Clear Vision Blueprint

Unlocking the Secrets to Healthy Eyes and Banishing Eye Problems

David Shaw

Copyright © (David Shaw) 2023. All rights reserved

The reproduction or duplication of this document is prohibited without the publisher's consent. Any electronic storage, transfer, or inclusion in a database is also prohibited. The document cannot be copied, scanned, faxed, or retained in part or in full without approval from the publisher or creator.

Table of Contents

Introduction
Chapter 1
Understanding Common Eye Conditions
    Importance of Early Detection and Treatment
Chapter 2
Eye Care Basics
    Healthy Habits for Maintaining Good Vision
    Importance of Regular Eye Exams
Chapter 3
Nourishing Your Eyes with a Balanced Diet
    Nutrients Essential for Eye Health
    Foods to Include in Your Diet for Optimal Eye Health
Chapter 4
Preventive Measures for Eye Problems
    Protecting Your Eyes from Harmful UV Radiation
    Preventing Eye Strain from Digital Devices
    Eye Safety Practices for Everyday Life
Chapter 5
Natural Remedies for Eye Health
    Soothing Eye Exercises and Relaxation Techniques
    Herbal Remedies for Common Eye Conditions
    Aromatherapy and Essential Oils for Eye Health
Chapter 6
Medications and Treatments for Eye Problems
    Over-the-Counter Eye Drops and Ointments

Prescription Medications for Specific Eye Conditions

Surgical Interventions for Corrective Eye Procedures

Chapter 7

Managing Specific Eye Conditions

Dry Eye Syndrome

Glaucoma

Cataracts

Chapter 8

Lifestyle Changes for Healthy Eyes

Tips for Reducing Eye Strain and Fatigue

Creating an Eye-Friendly Environment at Home and Work

Incorporating Exercise and Physical Activity for Eye Health

Chapter 9

Vision Care for Different Stages of Life

Eye Care for Children and Adolescents

Eye Health in Adults and the Aging Population

Addressing Vision Changes during Pregnancy

Chapter 10

Seeking Professional Help

Choosing an Optometrist or Ophthalmologist

Importance of Regular Check-ups and Follow-ups

Understanding Refractive Errors and Vision Correction

Vision correction options for refractive errors include

Conclusion

Introduction

Introducing the Clear Vision Blueprint: Unlocking the Secrets to Healthy Eyes and Banishing Eye Problems. Imagine a world where your eyesight is sharp, your vision crystal-clear, and your ocular health vibrant. No longer burdened by the constraints of eye problems, you embark on a journey towards optimal eye wellness. This revolutionary blueprint unveils the closely-guarded secrets to achieving and maintaining healthy eyes, offering a comprehensive roadmap to banish those pesky eye issues that have plagued you for far too long. With expert insights, proven strategies, and practical tips, the Clear Vision Blueprint empowers you to take control of your eye health, enabling you to see the world with renewed clarity and embrace the beauty that lies before you. It's time to unlock the hidden potential of your eyes and embark on a transformative path towards a future filled with clear vision and limitless possibilities.

Chapter 1

Understanding Common Eye Conditions

The focus is on familiarizing readers with some of the most prevalent eye conditions. It covers common eye problems such as refractive errors (e.g., nearsightedness, farsightedness, astigmatism), dry eye syndrome, glaucoma, cataracts, macular degeneration, and others. Each condition is briefly explained, including its causes, symptoms, and potential impact on vision.

Importance of Early Detection and Treatment

Emphasizes the significance of early detection and treatment in managing eye problems effectively. It highlights the benefits of regular eye exams in detecting eye conditions at their earliest stages when interventions can be most effective. The importance of promptly addressing any symptoms or changes in vision is also stressed, as it can prevent further deterioration and improve the chances of successful treatment.

By understanding common eye conditions and recognizing the importance of early detection and treatment, individuals can take proactive steps toward maintaining optimal eye health and seeking appropriate care when needed.

Chapter 2

Eye Care Basics

Eye care basics provides fundamental information on how to maintain good eye health through everyday practices and habits.

Healthy Habits for Maintaining Good Vision

Various habits and practices are discussed that contribute to maintaining good vision. It covers topics such as:

Proper Eye Hygiene: Tips for keeping your eyes clean and avoiding eye infections.

Balanced Diet: The importance of a nutritious diet rich in vitamins, minerals, and antioxidants for overall eye health.

Adequate Hydration: How staying hydrated benefits eye health.
Eye Protection: Tips for protecting your eyes from injury during sports, work, and daily activities.

Proper Lighting: The significance of adequate lighting conditions to prevent eye strain and discomfort.

Resting Your Eyes: The importance of regular breaks, especially during prolonged screen use, to reduce eye strain.

Avoiding Smoking: The harmful effects of smoking on eye health and the benefits of quitting.

By adopting healthy habits, individuals can promote and maintain good vision, reducing the risk of developing eye problems.

Importance of Regular Eye Exams

Emphasizes the significance of regular eye exams conducted by qualified eye care professionals. It covers the following aspects:

Detecting Eye Conditions: The ability of comprehensive eye exams to detect eye conditions, even in their early stages when symptoms may not be noticeable.

Vision Correction: Assessing the need for vision correction through glasses, contact lenses, or other means.

Eye Health Monitoring: Monitoring the overall health of the eyes, including the retina, optic nerve, and other vital structures.

Systemic Health Indicators: How eye exams can provide insights into an individual's overall health, as certain systemic conditions can manifest in the eyes.

Updating Prescriptions: The importance of updating prescriptions for glasses or contact lenses to maintain optimal visual acuity.

Regular eye exams play a crucial role in maintaining healthy eyes, preventing potential vision problems, and addressing any underlying issues promptly.

By following the eye care basics and prioritizing regular eye exams, individuals can take proactive measures to safeguard their vision and overall eye health.

Chapter 3

Nourishing Your Eyes with a Balanced Diet

Maintaining a balanced diet is crucial for promoting optimal eye health. By consuming a variety of nutrient-rich foods, you can provide your eyes with the essential vitamins and minerals they need to function properly.

Nutrients Essential for Eye Health

Certain nutrients play a key role in supporting and protecting your eyes. Consider including the following nutrients in your diet:

Vitamin A: Essential for good vision and overall eye health. It can be found in foods like carrots, sweet potatoes, spinach, and kale.

Omega-3 Fatty Acids: Help reduce the risk of age-related macular degeneration and dry eyes. Sources include fatty fish like salmon, mackerel, and trout, as well as flaxseeds and chia seeds.

Lutein and Zeaxanthin: Antioxidants that protect the eyes from harmful blue light and reduce the risk of macular degeneration and cataracts. Found in leafy green vegetables, broccoli, Brussels sprouts, and corn.

Vitamin C: An antioxidant that supports healthy blood vessels in the eyes and reduces the risk of cataracts. Citrus fruits, strawberries, bell peppers, and tomatoes are excellent sources.

Vitamin E: Protects cells in the eyes from damage caused by free radicals. Include foods like almonds, sunflower seeds, spinach, and avocados in your diet.

Zinc: Important for healthy vision and night vision. Sources include oysters, lean meats, poultry, beans, and nuts.

Antioxidants: Various antioxidants, such as beta-carotene (found in carrots, sweet potatoes, and apricots) and selenium (found in Brazil nuts and seafood), help protect the eyes from oxidative stress.

Foods to Include in Your Diet for Optimal Eye Health

To optimize your eye health, incorporate the following foods into your diet:

Leafy Green Vegetables: Spinach, kale, collard greens, and Swiss chard are rich in vitamins A, C, and E, as well as lutein and zeaxanthin.

Colorful Fruits and Vegetables: Carrots, oranges, berries, grapes, and bell peppers provide a range of eye-healthy nutrients.

Fatty Fish: Salmon, tuna, sardines, and trout are excellent sources of omega-3 fatty acids.

Nuts and Seeds: Almonds, walnuts, flaxseeds, and chia seeds offer omega-3 fatty acids and vitamin E.

Citrus Fruits: Oranges, grapefruits, and lemons are high in vitamin C.

Eggs: Rich in vitamins A, lutein, and zeaxanthin, eggs can contribute to good eye health.

Legumes: Kidney beans, lentils, and chickpeas provide zinc and other nutrients beneficial for eye health.

You can also consult with a healthcare professional or registered dietitian to tailor your diet based on your individual nutritional needs and any specific health conditions.

Chapter 4

Preventive Measures for Eye Problems

Preventing eye problems involves adopting various preventive measures and practices to maintain optimal eye health. This section covers important preventive measures for common eye issues.

Protecting Your Eyes from Harmful UV Radiation

Exposure to ultraviolet (UV) radiation can lead to various eye problems, including cataracts, macular degeneration, and photokeratitis (sunburn of the eye). Here are some preventive measures to protect your eyes from harmful UV radiation:

Wear Sunglasses: Choose sunglasses that block 100% of UVA and UVB rays. Opt for wraparound styles or those with large lenses to provide maximum coverage.

Use UV-Protective Contact Lenses: Consider using contact lenses that offer UV protection, in addition to wearing sunglasses.

Wear a Wide-Brimmed Hat: Pair your sunglasses with a wide-brimmed hat for added protection, especially during peak sunlight hours.

Preventing Eye Strain from Digital Devices

Extended use of digital devices can cause eye strain, dryness, blurred vision, and headaches. To prevent eye strain, consider the following measures:

Follow the 20-20-20 Rule: Every 20 minutes, take a 20-second break to look at something 20 feet away to reduce eye fatigue.

Adjust Display Settings: Optimize your device's brightness, contrast, and font size for comfortable viewing.

Blink Regularly: Remember to blink frequently to keep your eyes moist and prevent dryness.

Maintain Proper Posture: Sit at a comfortable distance from the screen, ensuring your eyes are level with the top of the monitor.

Use Blue Light Filters: Apply blue light filters or use specialized screen protectors to reduce the exposure to blue light emitted by digital screens.

Take Regular Breaks: Give your eyes periodic rest by taking breaks from screen time and engaging in other activities.

Eye Safety Practices for Everyday Life

Practicing good eye safety habits can prevent injuries and protect your eyes in various daily situations. Consider the following safety practices:

Use Protective Eyewear: When engaging in sports activities or working with tools, chemicals, or any potentially hazardous materials, wear appropriate safety glasses or goggles.

Be Cautious with Sharp Objects: Handle sharp objects with care to avoid eye injuries. Use appropriate protective eyewear when needed.

Practice Good Hygiene: Wash your hands thoroughly before touching your eyes to prevent the spread of infections.

Avoid Rubbing Your Eyes: Refrain from rubbing your eyes, as it can cause irritation and increase the risk of infections.

Keep Your Environment Clean: Maintain a clean and dust-free environment to minimize the risk of allergens and irritants affecting your eyes.

By following these preventive measures and practicing good eye safety, you can significantly reduce the risk of eye problems and maintain optimal eye health in your everyday life.

Chapter 5

Natural Remedies for Eye Health

Natural remedies can complement traditional eye care practices and promote overall eye health. This section covers some natural remedies that may be beneficial for maintaining healthy eyes.

Soothing Eye Exercises and Relaxation Techniques

Performing eye exercises and relaxation techniques can help alleviate eye strain and improve blood circulation around the eyes. Consider incorporating the following practices into your routine:

Palming: Rub your hands together to generate warmth and place them gently over your closed eyes. Relax and enjoy the darkness for a few minutes.

Eye Rolling: Slowly roll your eyes in a circular motion, both clockwise and counterclockwise. Repeat several times to relax the eye muscles.

Focus Shifting: Focus on a distant object for a few seconds, then shift your focus to something closer. Repeat this exercise to improve flexibility and focus adjustment.

Blinking: Rapidly blink your eyes for a few seconds to moisturize the surface and relieve dryness.

Herbal Remedies for Common Eye Conditions

Herbs have been used for centuries in traditional medicine to support eye health. It is important to consult with a healthcare professional before using any herbal remedies, especially if you have pre-existing eye conditions or are taking medications. Here are some herbs commonly associated with eye health:

Bilberry: Known for its antioxidant properties, bilberry may help improve night vision and promote healthy blood vessels in the eyes.

Eyebright: Traditionally used to alleviate eye irritation and inflammation, eyebright is believed to have a soothing effect on the eyes.

Ginkgo Biloba: This herb is thought to improve blood flow to the eyes and protect against age-related eye diseases.

Calendula: With anti-inflammatory properties, calendula may assist in relieving eye irritations and promoting overall eye health.

Aromatherapy and Essential Oils for Eye Health

Aromatherapy, using essential oils derived from plants, can provide a calming effect and potentially support eye health. It's important to dilute essential oils properly and avoid direct contact with the eyes. Some essential oils that may be used in aromatherapy for eye health include:

Lavender: Known for its soothing properties, lavender oil can help relax the eye muscles and promote a sense of calm.

Roman Chamomile: With anti-inflammatory effects, chamomile oil may assist in reducing eye inflammation and irritation.

Cypress: Cypress oil is believed to improve circulation and support healthy blood vessels in the eyes.

Always ensure that you are using high-quality essential oils, and consult with a qualified aromatherapist or healthcare professional for proper usage and safety guidelines.

While natural remedies can provide additional support for eye health, they should not replace professional medical advice or treatment. It's important to consult with an eye care specialist for any persistent or serious eye conditions.

Chapter 6

Medications and Treatments for Eye Problems

When it comes to treating various eye problems, different medications and treatments are available. This section explores some common options for addressing eye issues.

Over-the-Counter Eye Drops and Ointments

Over-the-counter (OTC) eye drops and ointments can provide relief for certain eye conditions. It's important to read and follow the instructions carefully and consult with a healthcare professional if symptoms persist or worsen. Some types of OTC eye drops and ointments include:

Artificial Tears: Lubricating eye drops that can alleviate dryness and provide temporary relief from eye discomfort.

Allergy Eye Drops: Antihistamine or mast cell stabilizer eye drops that can help relieve itching, redness, and other symptoms associated with eye allergies.

Redness Relievers: Eye drops that temporarily reduce redness, typically by constricting blood vessels in the eyes. These should be used for short-term relief only.

Prescription Medications for Specific Eye Conditions

For more severe or chronic eye conditions, prescription medications may be necessary. Some common prescription medications for specific eye conditions include:

Antibiotics: Prescribed to treat bacterial eye infections such as conjunctivitis (pink eye) or corneal ulcers.

Antiviral Drugs: Used to treat viral eye infections, such as those caused by herpes simplex or varicella-zoster viruses.

Anti-inflammatory Medications: Can help reduce inflammation in the eyes caused by conditions like uveitis or ocular inflammation.

Glaucoma Medications: Eye drops or oral medications prescribed to lower intraocular pressure and manage glaucoma.

Corticosteroids: Prescribed to manage various eye conditions, including allergic conjunctivitis, uveitis, or inflammation after eye surgery.

Surgical Interventions for Corrective Eye Procedures

In certain cases, surgical interventions may be necessary to address specific eye conditions or to correct vision problems. Some common surgical procedures include:

Cataract Surgery: Involves removing the clouded lens of the eye and replacing it with an artificial intraocular lens (IOL) to restore clear vision.

LASIK (Laser-Assisted In Situ Keratomileusis): A refractive surgery procedure that uses a laser to reshape the cornea and correct nearsightedness, farsightedness, and astigmatism.

PRK (Photorefractive Keratectomy): Similar to LASIK, PRK is a refractive surgery that uses a laser to reshape the cornea. It is often recommended for individuals with thinner corneas or specific corneal conditions.

Retinal Surgery: Various surgical procedures are performed to repair retinal detachments, macular holes, or other conditions affecting the retina.

Glaucoma Surgery: Several surgical options are available to lower intraocular pressure and manage glaucoma when medications alone are insufficient.

These surgical interventions are performed by qualified ophthalmologists and require careful evaluation and discussion with a healthcare professional to determine the most suitable treatment option for each individual.

It's important to consult with a healthcare professional or ophthalmologist for a proper diagnosis, personalized treatment plan, and to discuss the potential risks and benefits associated with specific medications or surgical procedures.

Chapter 7

Managing Specific Eye Conditions

This section focuses on three specific eye conditions, including their causes, symptoms, and available treatment options.

Dry Eye Syndrome

Dry Eye Syndrome occurs when the eyes do not produce enough tears or when the tears evaporate too quickly.

Causes:
- Aging

- Hormonal changes
- Certain medications
- Environmental factors
- Underlying health conditions.

Symptoms:
- Dryness, itchiness, or a gritty sensation in the eyes.
- Excessive tearing or watery eyes as a reflex response.
- Redness and irritation
- Blurred vision or sensitivity to light.

Treatment

Artificial Tears: Over-the-counter lubricating eye drops can provide temporary relief.

Prescription Eye Drops: Medications that help increase tear production or reduce inflammation in the eyes.

Warm Compresses: Applying warm compresses to the eyes can help open oil glands and improve tear quality.

Lifestyle Modifications: Avoiding dry environments, using a humidifier, wearing sunglasses outdoors, and taking breaks from digital screens can help alleviate symptoms.

In severe cases, additional treatments such as punctal plugs (to block tear drainage) or therapies like intense pulsed light (IPL) may be recommended.

Glaucoma

Glaucoma is a group of eye diseases characterized by damage to the optic nerve, often associated with increased intraocular pressure (IOP). If left untreated, it can lead to permanent vision loss.

Causes: The exact cause is unknown, high IOP is a significant risk factor.

Symptoms: It may not be noticeable until later stages.

Gradual loss of peripheral vision (most common in open-angle glaucoma).
Tunnel vision or narrowed field of vision.
Blurred vision or halos around lights.
Severe eye pain, headaches, or nausea (in acute angle-closure glaucoma).

Treatment:

Eye Drops

Medications that lower intraocular pressure by reducing the production of fluid in the eye or improving drainage.

Oral Medications

In some cases, oral medications may be prescribed to lower IOP.

Laser Therapy

Procedures like selective laser trabeculoplasty (SLT) or laser peripheral iridotomy (LPI) can improve fluid drainage or reduce IOP.

Surgical Interventions

Trabeculectomy, glaucoma drainage implants, or minimally invasive glaucoma surgeries (MIGS) may be considered for more advanced cases.

Cataracts

Cataracts refer to the clouding of the eye's natural lens, leading to vision impairment.

Causes:
- Age-related changes.
- Injury.
- Certain medications, underlying medical conditions.

Symptoms:
- Blurred
- Hazy, cloudy vision
- Sensitivity to glare, particularly from bright lights
- Difficulty seeing at night or in low-light conditions
- Fading or yellowing of colors
- Frequent changes in glasses or contact lens prescriptions

Treatments: The primary treatment for cataracts is surgical removal.

Cataract surgery involves removing the cloudy lens and replacing it with an artificial intraocular lens (IOL) to restore clear vision.

Advanced surgical techniques, such as laser-assisted cataract surgery, can further enhance the precision and outcomes of the procedure.

It's important to consult with an eye care specialist or ophthalmologist for accurate diagnosis, personalized treatment plans, and to discuss the potential risks and benefits associated with specific treatments or surgeries.

Chapter 8

Lifestyle Changes for Healthy Eyes

Taking care of your overall health and incorporating certain lifestyle changes can contribute to maintaining healthy eyes. This section covers various tips and practices for promoting eye health.

Tips for Reducing Eye Strain and Fatigue

Prolonged use of digital devices and other activities that require intense visual concentration can cause eye strain and fatigue. Consider the following tips to reduce strain and keep your eyes refreshed:

Take Regular Breaks: Follow the 20-20-20 rule – every 20 minutes, take a 20-second break to look at something 20 feet away.

Blink Frequently: Blinking helps moisten the eyes and prevent dryness. Be conscious of blinking regularly, especially during focused tasks.

Adjust Lighting: Ensure that your workspace has appropriate lighting. Avoid harsh glare or overly dim lighting that strains the eyes.

Maintain Proper Distance: Position your computer screen or reading material at a comfortable distance to reduce the need for excessive eye focusing or strain.

Use Corrective Lenses: If you require glasses or contact lenses, make sure your prescription is up to date to avoid unnecessary eye strain.

Consider Blue Light Filters: Apply blue light filters or use specialized screen protectors to minimize exposure to blue light emitted by digital screens.

Creating an Eye-Friendly Environment at Home and Work

Optimizing your environment for eye health can contribute to long-term well-being. Consider the following practices to create an eye-friendly environment:

Proper Lighting: Use adjustable lighting sources and avoid overly bright or harsh lighting that can strain the eyes.

Reduce Glare: Position your computer or other screens to minimize glare from windows or overhead lights. Consider using anti-glare screen filters.

Monitor Placement: Position your computer monitor or screen slightly below eye level to reduce strain on the neck and eyes.

Keep the Environment Clean: Maintain cleanliness to minimize dust and allergens that can irritate the eyes.

Maintain Humidity: Use a humidifier in dry environments to prevent dry eyes. Keep humidity levels balanced for optimal eye comfort.

Incorporating Exercise and Physical Activity for Eye Health

Regular physical activity and exercise can promote overall health, including eye health. Consider the following activities to support eye health:

Cardiovascular Exercises: Engage in aerobic exercises such as walking, running, swimming, or cycling to improve blood circulation, including to the eyes.

Eye Exercises: Incorporate specific eye exercises to help improve eye muscle strength and flexibility. These may include focusing on near and far objects, eye rolling, or palming.

Yoga and Tai Chi: These gentle, low-impact exercises can help reduce eye strain, improve circulation, and promote relaxation.

Outdoor Activities: Spend time outdoors to benefit from natural light and encourage distance vision. This can help reduce the risk of myopia progression in children and adolescents.

Remember to consult with a healthcare professional before starting any new exercise routine, especially if you have underlying health conditions.

By adopting these lifestyle changes and incorporating practices that reduce eye strain, create an eye-friendly environment, and promote physical activity, you can support your eye health and overall well-being.

Chapter 9

Vision Care for Different Stages of Life

Eye health needs can vary across different stages of life. This section explores vision care considerations for children and adolescents, adults and the aging population, as well as addressing vision changes during pregnancy.

Eye Care for Children and Adolescents

Children and adolescents require proper vision care to support their overall development and academic performance. Consider the following aspects:

Regular Eye Exams: Schedule comprehensive eye exams for children, starting around 6 months of age, and then at age 3, before entering school, and periodically throughout their school years.

Vision Correction: If needed, provide children with appropriate glasses or contact lenses to correct refractive errors (nearsightedness, farsightedness, or astigmatism).

Protective Eyewear: Encourage the use of protective eyewear during sports or activities that pose a risk of eye injury.

Balanced Screen Time: Help children maintain a healthy balance between screen time and other activities, ensuring they take breaks and practice good visual habits.

Proper Lighting: Ensure that the lighting in their study areas or when using digital devices is adequate to reduce eye strain.

Regular eye exams during childhood are essential for early detection and intervention of vision problems.

Eye Health in Adults and the Aging Population

As adults age, the risk of developing age-related eye conditions increases. Consider the following aspects for maintaining good eye health:

Regular Eye Exams: Schedule comprehensive eye exams every 1-2 years, or as recommended by an eye care professional, to detect and manage age-related eye conditions such as cataracts, glaucoma, or age-related macular degeneration (AMD).

Manage Chronic Conditions: Maintain overall health and manage chronic conditions like diabetes or hypertension, which can impact eye health.

Maintain Healthy Lifestyle: Adopt a balanced diet rich in fruits, vegetables, and omega-3 fatty acids. Maintain a healthy weight and engage in regular exercise to support overall well-being, including eye health.

Protect from UV Radiation: Wear sunglasses with UV protection when outdoors to reduce the risk of cataracts and other eye conditions caused by excessive sun exposure.

Quit Smoking: Smoking increases the risk of several eye conditions, including cataracts and AMD.

Quitting smoking can significantly improve eye health.

Monitor Medications: Be aware of the potential side effects of medications on eye health and discuss any concerns with healthcare professionals.

Addressing Vision Changes during Pregnancy

Pregnancy can bring temporary changes to vision due to hormonal fluctuations and fluid retention. Consider the following aspects during pregnancy:

Hormonal Changes: Pregnancy hormones may cause dry eyes or changes in visual acuity. Use artificial tears to alleviate dryness and consult an eye care professional if significant changes in vision occur.

Gestational Diabetes: Pregnant women with gestational diabetes have an increased risk of developing diabetic retinopathy. Regular prenatal care and monitoring of blood glucose levels are crucial.

Preeclampsia This condition characterized by high blood pressure can affect vision. Regular blood pressure checkups and monitoring for visual disturbances are important.

Safety Precautions: Use caution when applying medications or eye drops during pregnancy. Consult with healthcare professionals to ensure the safety of any treatments.

Regular prenatal care, maintaining overall health, and promptly addressing any vision changes or concerns are key during pregnancy.

Remember, the information provided here is general in nature. It's important to consult with an eye care professional or healthcare provider for personalized advice and recommendations based on individual circumstances.

Chapter 10

Seeking Professional Help

When it comes to maintaining optimal eye health and addressing vision concerns, seeking professional help from optometrists or ophthalmologists is crucial. This section covers the importance of choosing the right eye care professional, the significance of regular check-ups and follow-ups, and understanding refractive errors and vision correction.

Choosing an Optometrist or Ophthalmologist

Both optometrists and ophthalmologists play essential roles in eye care, but their areas of expertise differ. Consider the following when choosing the right eye care professional:

Optometrist: Optometrists are primary eye care providers who specialize in performing comprehensive eye exams, diagnosing and managing common eye conditions, prescribing glasses or contact lenses, and providing pre- and post-operative care for certain eye surgeries. They may also provide vision therapy for certain conditions.

Ophthalmologist: Ophthalmologists are medical doctors (MDs) or doctors of osteopathic medicine (DOs) who specialize in eye care and surgery. They can diagnose and treat eye diseases, perform surgeries (such as cataract surgery or LASIK), prescribe medications, and provide comprehensive eye care.

Consider your specific needs and the nature of your eye condition to determine whether you need the expertise of an optometrist or an ophthalmologist. In some cases, both professionals may work together for comprehensive eye care.

Importance of Regular Check-ups and Follow-ups

Regular eye check-ups are essential for maintaining optimal eye health and detecting potential problems early. Consider the following reasons for regular check-ups and follow-ups:

Early Detection: Eye conditions often develop gradually and may not have noticeable symptoms in the early stages. Regular check-ups can help detect problems before they progress and cause irreversible damage.

Vision Correction: Regular eye exams ensure that your prescription for glasses or contact lenses is up to date, allowing for clear and comfortable vision.

Monitoring Eye Conditions: If you have an existing eye condition, regular follow-ups with your eye care professional will help monitor the condition's progression, adjust treatments as needed, and address any concerns.

Overall Health Assessment: Eye exams can also provide insights into your overall health. Some systemic conditions, such as diabetes or hypertension, can be detected through an eye examination.

Understanding Refractive Errors and Vision Correction

Refractive errors are common vision problems that occur when the shape of the eye prevents light from focusing properly on the retina, leading to blurred vision. Common refractive errors include:

Nearsightedness (Myopia): Distant objects appear blurry, while close objects are clearer.

Farsightedness (Hyperopia): Close objects appear blurry, while distant objects are clearer.

Astigmatism: Blurred or distorted vision at all distances due to an irregularly shaped cornea or lens.

Vision correction options for refractive errors include

Glasses: Prescription glasses consist of lenses specifically designed to compensate for the refractive error and provide clear vision.

Contact Lenses: These thin, curved lenses are placed directly on the eye's surface to correct refractive errors. Different types, such as daily disposables or extended wear lenses, are available to suit individual needs.

Refractive Surgery: Surgical procedures like LASIK, PRK, or implantable lenses can reshape the cornea or replace the eye's natural lens to correct refractive errors permanently.

Consult with your eye care professional to determine the most suitable vision correction option based on your visual needs, lifestyle, and eye health.

Regular eye check-ups, appropriate professional guidance, and understanding your vision needs are key to maintaining optimal eye health and addressing vision concerns effectively.

Conclusion

In conclusion, taking care of your eyes and maintaining optimal eye health is crucial for overall well-being and quality of life. By understanding common eye conditions, the importance of early detection and treatment, and implementing preventive measures, you can proactively protect your vision.

Recap of Key Points
Throughout this guide, we have covered various aspects of eye care. Here is a recap of the key points discussed:

Understanding common eye conditions: Familiarize yourself with common eye conditions, their causes, symptoms, and treatment options.

Importance of early detection and treatment: Regular eye exams are vital for early detection of eye problems, which allows for prompt treatment and better outcomes.

Developing healthy habits: Adopt healthy habits such as maintaining a balanced diet, getting regular exercise, reducing eye strain from digital devices, and practicing good eye safety measures.

Nourishing your eyes with a balanced diet: Include foods rich in nutrients essential for eye health, such as omega-3 fatty acids, vitamins C and E, lutein, zeaxanthin, and zinc.

Preventive measures for eye problems: Protect your eyes from harmful UV radiation, prevent eye strain from digital devices, and practice eye safety in everyday life.

Natural remedies for eye health: Explore soothing eye exercises, relaxation techniques, herbal remedies, aromatherapy, and essential oils to support eye health.

Medications and treatments for eye problems: Understand over-the-counter eye drops, prescription medications, and surgical interventions available for treating specific eye conditions.

Managing specific eye conditions: Learn about managing dry eye syndrome, glaucoma, cataracts, and other common eye conditions through lifestyle changes, medications, or surgical interventions.

Lifestyle changes for healthy eyes: Implement tips to reduce eye strain and fatigue, create an eye-friendly environment at home and work, and incorporate exercise and physical activity for optimal eye health.

Vision care for different stages of life: Consider the specific eye care needs for children and adolescents, adults and the aging population, as well as addressing vision changes during pregnancy.

Seeking professional help: Choose the right eye care professional, schedule regular check-ups and follow-ups, and understand refractive errors and vision correction options.

Developing an Eye Care Routine
To maintain optimal eye health, it's important to develop a consistent eye

care routine. Here are some steps to consider:

Schedule regular eye exams: Follow the recommended frequency for comprehensive eye exams based on your age, existing conditions, and professional advice.

Practice good eye hygiene: Wash your hands before touching your eyes, remove eye makeup properly, and avoid rubbing your eyes excessively.

Follow a balanced diet: Incorporate foods rich in eye-healthy nutrients, such as leafy greens, citrus fruits, fish, nuts, and seeds.

Protect your eyes: Wear sunglasses with UV protection, use safety eyewear when necessary, and follow proper eye safety practices in your daily activities.

Manage chronic conditions: If you have underlying health conditions like diabetes or hypertension, work closely with your healthcare team to manage them effectively, as they can impact eye health.

Practice healthy screen habits: Take regular breaks when using digital devices, adjust screen settings for comfort, and maintain proper posture to reduce eye strain.

Maintain overall health: Adopt a healthy lifestyle that includes regular exercise, adequate sleep, and managing stress levels, as these factors contribute to overall eye health.

Follow professional recommendations: Adhere to prescribed medications, vision correction options, or treatment plans provided by your eye care professional.

Empowering Yourself to Maintain Optimal Eye Health

Empower yourself to take control of your eye health by staying informed and proactive. Here are some ways to empower yourself:

Stay informed: Stay updated on the latest developments in eye care, advancements in treatments, and lifestyle practices for maintaining optimal eye health.

Educate yourself: Learn about common eye conditions, symptoms to watch for, and the importance of early detection and treatment.

Ask questions: During eye exams or consultations, don't hesitate to ask your eye care professional about any concerns, treatment options, or lifestyle recommendations.

Advocate for your eye health: Be an active participant in your eye care by following professional advice, practicing healthy habits, and seeking timely care when needed.

Spread awareness: Share your knowledge and experiences with family, friends, and the community to raise awareness about the importance of eye health.

Take action today to prioritize your eye health and embark on a journey of lifelong visual wellness.